Faces of Uterine Fibroids

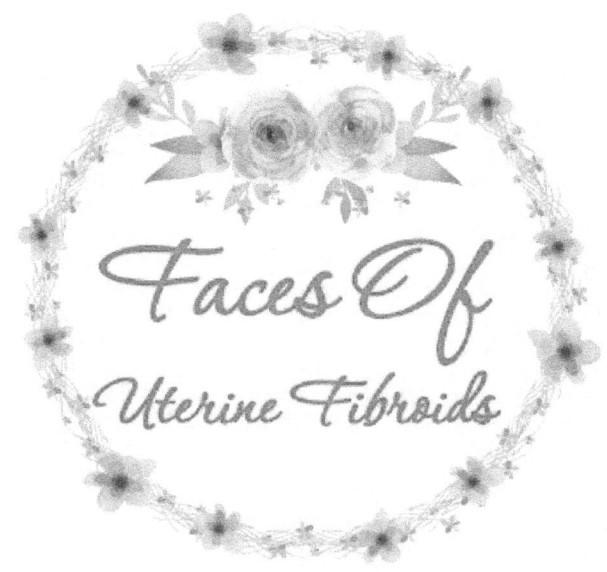

Untold Stories of A Woman's Biggest Secrets

Compilation by

Martine M. Mayas

Co-Authored with:

Dr. Stephanie Shanklin, Patrice Ross, Andrea E. Monroe

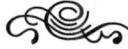

The events in this book actually happened.

A Compilation of International Women sharing their stories and experiences of uterine fibroids before, and after surgery.

Uterine Fibroids

Fibroids are muscular tumors that grow in the wall of the uterus (womb). Fibroids are almost always benign (not cancerous). Not all women with fibroids have symptoms. Women who do have symptoms often find fibroids hard to live with. Some have pain and heavy menstrual bleeding. Treatment for uterine fibroids depends on your symptoms.

~ www.womenshealth.gov

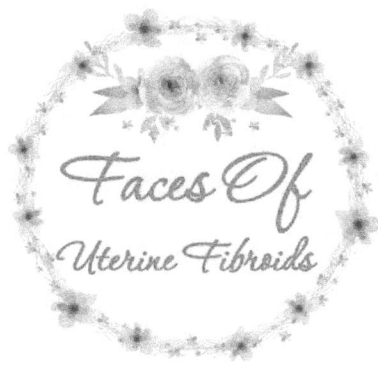

This Book is dedicated to all Fibroid Warriors,

Please keep in mind that uterine fibroids is a condition, not a disease. It is a conversation which needs to be discussed on all levels in all industries. It is imperative to speak and allow others to know of uterine fibroids for awareness, education, and research. You cannot continue to suffer in silence with a condition that is detrimental to your mind, body, and soul. Be sure to put shame, and embarrassment behind you, as you indulge into the shared stories of a few different women, just like you. You are not alone. I know the signs and symptoms of uterine fibroids are painful, but we all must learn to release our pain by accepting our condition, embracing the struggles from within in order to release our upsets for a better tomorrow.

Contents

Foreword

"When we are empowered, we make better decisions"

VLADIMIRE CALIXTE

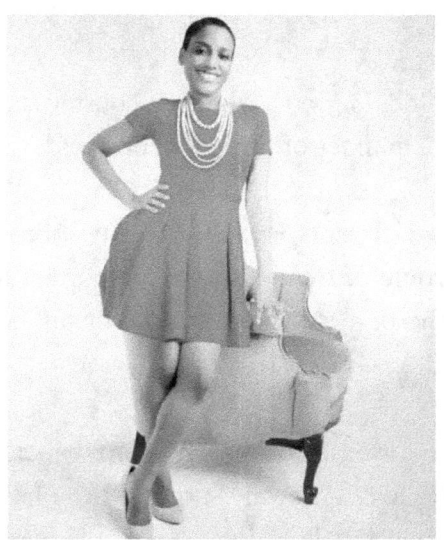

My journey with uterine fibroids dates back to my early twenties. As I think back, it's something that I didn't know at the time. I was experiencing severe cramping and heavy bleeding during my menses. However, I just figured that it was normal. Over the years, the fibroids just continue to grow and cause other concerns, unbeknownst to me.

Fast forward, married with an unbridled joy of expectation of having children to be dismayed, month after month and year after year.

What became apparent were the constant 'flooding' through my clothes, painful intercourse, severe cramping and heavy bleeding, frequent urination, back pain, and infertility. Until several pelvic ultrasounds later detected over 30 fibroids.

My infertility was the most painful for me to process emotionally. Because most of the fibroids were nestled in my endometrium (the inside lining of the uterus), it was impossible to conceive. Thus, three years of not knowing whether or not my husband and I would ever be able to have children.

By the grace of God, I found a wonderful obstetrician/gynecologist who recommended a number of treatment options.

Because of the size and location of my fibroids, I chose a myomectomy as a route of treatment. It is important to note that the myomectomy was the best treatment option for me because I deeply desired to have children.

I underwent the myomectomy, where my doctor removed 32 fibroids. Yes, 32 fibroids!! After my surgery, I still had some fibroids left that were too small for detection. As such, I made a decision to change my diet and exercise routine, which helped me tremendously.

Today, I am fibroids free!

I had my surgery in February of 2005 and my husband and I conceived in February of 2006. God blessed us with our daughter and three years, thereafter, our son.

I am a big proponent that when we are empowered, we make better decisions. As such, my advice to other women is to discuss all of the different treatment options available with your gynecologist – the most important thing is having all the facts, understanding your body and considering the best options for your personal situation.

If I could talk to my younger self, I would advise to seek medical assistance much sooner.

Lastly, if you are living with uterine fibroids, please know that you are not alone. Please don't suffer in silence! Silence will keep in you a place that doesn't serve you well, physically, emotionally and spiritually.

Vladimire Calixte, MA, CRC, LMHC
Celebrity Therapist
New York, New York, 2017
www.LifeRebuilding.com

About the Author

MARTINE M. MAYAS
I AM A FIBROID WARRIOR

As a Fibroid Warrior for 21 years, I am taking responsibility to share my story for this condition. On November 16, 2016, I had an open myomectomy to remove multiple uterine fibroids. Thank God all went well. Now, I am ready to speak out and help others by creating this anthology by women for women concerning uterine fibroids.

This anthology is called Faces of Uterine Fibroids. It's a compilation of short stories of women sharing their journeys before and after surgery concerning uterine fibroids.
The goal is to give hope, courage and inspiration to those suffering.

Martine M. Mayas was born in 1976 in New York to Haitian parents, Jocelyne Mayas and Frantz Mayas. Martine is a Natural Hair Enthusiast and an International Best Selling Author who shares her personal life experiences, style, poise, etiquette, class and sophistication with the world. Contact Martine at email: mindhearthairbodysoul@gmail.com.

What People are saying...

This book is so important to bring awareness to a topic that is so common and so many women are suffering in silence. I am happy that these stories are coming to light. Martine Mayas has created a community of healers with this book. As the writers share their stories, it will bring comfort, education, and understanding to many women who are experiencing fibroids. — *Yvelette Stines, author of Vernon the Vegetable Man and Be Calm: 31 Mindful Affirmations and Reflections for Living a Peaceful Life*

Martine Mayas and "The Faces of Uterine Fibroids" has been one of the best things that has not only happened to me but to the entire fibroid community. As a uterine fibroid warrior myself, I appreciate Martine for giving so much of herself and sharing important health tips as well as leaving an open forum for all women to discuss their issues, concerns & journeys. In becoming a licensed massage therapist, I love using all natural health products such as essential oils, but I can never learn enough about this issue and I continue to learn because of this extraordinary project by an extraordinary woman. *Thank you Martine!* ~*Angel L. Varner, LMT*

What People are saying...

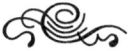

Faces of Uterine Fibroids by Martine Mayas is a chilling vision of things to come that will leave you mentally casting the movie adaption. I once ask a woman how many months is she, and when she replied she has Fibroids, I knew I needed to read this book. Do yourself and me a favor call up the New York Times and politely ask if they could please help you understand why they only gave the author's last Book three stars despite its obvious brilliance, and could they perhaps run a correction and apology. *~Chief Social Media Officer, Chef J. Juvon*

Are You Ready to have a conversation about Fibroids? Ready or not, women are no longer ashamed of sharing their stories. We all heal and overcome by the power our testimony! Faces of Uterine Fibroids is a journey of healing and breaking the chains of shame so women can be whole again! *~ Andrenee Boothe ~Master Life Strategist, Author and Blogger*

Stories that need to be shared! Uterine fibroids are commonalities shared among many women, yet one of the least likely topics to be discussed over branch; I am delighted that Martine Mayas has authored a unique composition to not only raise awareness but unity as well. I am sure these stories will be passed down from generation to generation of women, whispering a message in each chapter to the reader, that they are not alone. *~ Darlene A. Anderson ~Darlene's Utopia Committed to Helping you Discover Your Utopian Within*

I want to give a huge shout out and congratulations to the amazing Martine Mayas on her book, Faces of Uterine Fibroids. Martine is taking the initiative to be a strong voice to bring awareness to Uterine Fibroids and the struggles of women that are suffering with the condition. She is making sure that women that are struggling with this condition know that they are not alone and there is hope. *~ LeaAnn Fuller, Life Coach, Fuller Life, LLC Find your Power, Passion, and Purpose*

Kudos to Martine, for creating this platform, and allowing women to share their thoughts and feelings of living with Fibroid's.This is a touchy subject, as many suffer in silence. I'm sure bringing this subject to life is going to help spread the word what is helpful for those who suffer *~ Shequita Lee Author, Speaker & Social Media Coach*

Martine is the real deal, passionate, organized and giving. She is a supportive woman of herself and other women on their journey. She stops nothing of short with her beautiful determination. Definitely no "fitting in a box here" for Martine. This book Faces of Uterine Fibroids will serve so many on a lot of different levels *~ Kim Boudreau Smith ~ Life Coach, Author and Blogger*

What People are saying...

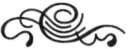

I salute Martine Maya's for her transparency regarding her fight with Uterine Fibroids. Martine is authentic and her story of being a Uterine Fibroid Warrior is an inspiration to women across the country. Faces of Uterine Fibroids provides education, support and hope. Anyone suffering from this condition will find comfort in the stories and testimonies shared. *~ Monique Denton-Davis, Founder and CEO, Embrace Your CAKE, LLC*

I want to say congratulations to Author Martine Mayas for moving forward with the mission to start a community to cater to women in pain, the most important part of her journey is that she feels what they feel and understand that hiding the pain only leads to more pain and hurt. As she moves forward with this project for communities, I know people will be blessed and encourage to speak out. More and more women are deciding not to hide behind the pain any more, but have nowhere to go leaving them isolated and lonely, but now you have a community of women that want to hold your hand and walk with you on that journey. I want to salute you Martine Mayas for creating that platform and ladies welcome to deliverance it's time to heal together! *~ Dr. Serena Washington, Your Coachsulting Advisor*

As the number of women living with fibroid tumors is growing each year, education is very important. Due to lack of knowledge about fibriods, many women are living with the tumors unknowingly, while others rely on a hysterectomy as a cure. Education about the diagnosis, as well as the treatments is vital. *~Tammy Jurnett-Lewis*

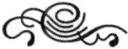

It's been said that 7 out of 10 women will battle with fibroids by age 50. This is a pretty high number and I know that this can be hard for a lot of women to deal with by themselves. Martine Mayas is a Warrior & truly an Unstoppable Woman. Being a survivor of Uterine fibroids she has now created a Movement and a space for women to not only come together who battle with this, but to be able to share their stories with a world and other women who are suffering in silence. I truly admire Martine's tenacity and determination to not give up on herself or the women that she has been called to serve on this journey. This Movement is life-changing and will create more women across the Nation who will finally speak up, stand in their truth and allow their voices to be heard.. I salute you. *~Shavannah Moore ~ Entrepreneur, Empowerment Speaker, Author*

The incredible women who have come together with Martine Mayas through her own epic journey puts Faces of Uterine Fibroids front and center. The stories bring a chill, and harshness that now Hollywood movie producers or ghost writers could do justice. For Martine and these women, the journey is empowering, thought provoking and raw with emotions that you can't help, but want to hug these women. Martine's insights to this very of topic of women's issues surpasses the most. She is a force to be heard. Women who suffer from Uterine Fibroids rise up, for she is in your corner, she's your voice, your beacon of hope and understanding. Powerful, gut-wrenching. Love and Compassion, this a MUST READ for all women! *~Patty Loehn-Beach, Engagement & Impact Coach, It's Possible PR*

What People are saying...

An excellent book that shines a light on an issue plaguing women of all ages. *~ Gaboy Jupiter, Nurse Practitioner*

Faces of Uterine Fibroids by Martine Mayas is an intimate look at a common problem that so many women face in silence and solitude. Martine has fiercley tackled this chronic condition with tact and grace with the end result a healing and hopeful mindset for women. Bravo Martine!   *~ Karen A. Thomas, Etiquette Educator, Speaker, Author, Trainer*

As the publisher, I take great pride of this influential compilation "Faces of Uterine Fibroids" by #1 International Author Martine M. Mayas. When Martine reached out in 2016, I believe it was just a few weeks before her surgery, and then again she reached out the day after to let us know everything had gone well…you could hear her excitement in her voice, it was so beautiful. At that moment, I just knew her story must be heard! Yet her journey isn't over, I know her story all too well, "somethings as women we don't talk about", until now, I Thank -You, Martine M. Maya's, and all her Co-Authors you have given all women a voice, a movement to raise awareness to all women living with Uterine Fibroids. *~ IrenePro, CEO, Publisher, Executive Creative Director, We are Beautiful Magazine©*

It's Time to make our Voices Heard!

~ We are Beautiful Magazine©

Acknowledgments

Congratulations are in order to all contributing authors. This book could not have come into existence without you.

Thank you for sharing your deepest experiencing with us for the betterment of bringing hope, courage, and inspiration to others.

We are thankful to our Prayer Warriors for their commitment in being of service for our book journey and movement.

Special thanks to all contributing blurbs for showing interest in Faces of Uterine Fibroids Movement.

Our deepest gratitude goes to you, our readers for your commencement of spreading awareness for the condition of uterine fibroids.

Maintain your focus, mind your business. Be your rescue. Gain freedom. Be free. Be the Master of your own life, like Master Jesus Christ.

~ Andrenee Boothe, Author, Blogger, Master Life Strategist

The Day of My Deliverance

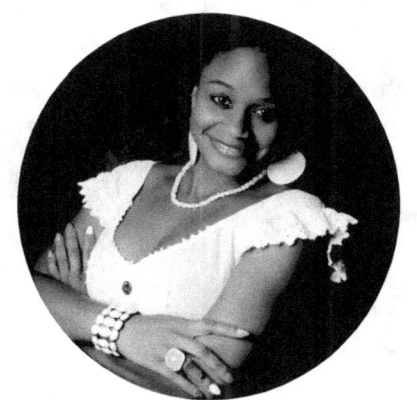

BY MARTINE M. MAYAS

I remember the days when I used to be a "live ice-crusher", craving and eating ice all day and night. It was so bad that I used to go bed with a cup of ice placed on my night table because I would definitely drink that ice-cold water in the middle of the night. I remember the days when I used to be mentally, physically and emotionally weak because I suffered from poor blood circulation due to being severely anemic with a blood count of five on the regular. I remember the days when I used to panic from fears of everything due to anxiety. I remember the days when I used to battle with confusion, and doubt due to lack of confidence because of a big secret held inside of me. Yes, indeed, I remember those days. Although I tried my best to be positive, it just never seemed to be enough because I always felt that I had a setback. The setback of being limited in my life. The setback of not having options because of diagnoses being put on my life and my condition. I remember growing up and being told that I was different, which was obvious to me, but never clarified because my condition was invisible. I always looked phenomenal on the outside. Everyone always loved my look and my style without knowing that my issues were inside of me. I lived my life in a bubble, hoping that the best love relationship would come and rescue me from this horrible condition, in order for me to move forward. But, unfortunately, that did not happen. Twenty-one years later, I find myself facing the possibility of having surgery because my options now had new limitations.

After seeing a network of doctors, one physician deliberately told me that I needed to have surgery for the benefit of living. A blood count of five was not something that my body could further sustain. So, I had two options, either a open myomectomy, which is the removal of uterine fibroids, or a hysterectomy which is the removal of the uterus, which will prevent uterine fibroids from returning after surgery. Since I did not have any children, physicians were always afraid to operate on me due to the difficulties of my case. Hence, the reason why they never even suggested treatment options with me. I educated myself by simply researching on my condition, trying herbal remedies at my own risk. That is how I survived for twenty-one years with multiple uterine fibroids on the inside and outside of my uterus, growing like multiple fetuses in my womb. The life I lived was heavy because of the load I carried inside of me. Wherever I went, they were always with me, during the good times, and the bad times. I came to a point where I accepted them, and deliberately shared my condition with a few, but that only resulted in them thinking and saying that I was crazy. So, on a positive note, I owned the craziness being labeled on me, and my life by others based on my condition with uterine fibroids. I made crazy look so beautiful with great boldness, hope, courage, and inspiration. Although they labeled me, they were always intrigued to learn, and know more of me. So, I kept pushing with faith. My beliefs that my deliverance was near was all I needed. My complaints and concerns were a dialogue shared between me and my God. That is when I was assured that God was enough. Listen to God's calling, and all will come around. That is exactly what happened.

Twenty-one years later, I find myself partnering with a physician who took my case, followed my condition, prepared me for an open myomectomy in order to remove those demons from the inside and outside of my uterus. He assured me with much precaution that my condition was deplorable but yet durable for a miracle with God's grace. The willingness to proceed was on me. After careful educated thoughts, I decided to go through with my decision as plan to remove these uterine fibroids in order to advance my life. At the age of forty years old, I was just at thetip of the iceberg to make it of a turning point in my life. The question and concern were "Do I want to have the possibility to conceive or not?" That was really the main concern since I don't have children. As I look back into my life, I am the only child of both of my parents and left with one parent since my father passed away three months after my birth. So, at that point, I truly did not believe that I would be robbed from more possibilities, my faith denounced that I've dealt with enough for a while. Why not open myself up to new possibilities by being intentional? You never know which doors may open for you? That is how I plunged into surgery on November 16, 2016, a date I will never forget. November 16, 2016, was indeed the day of my deliverance. I could not wait for that day to come. The more I prayed, the more I saw myself as the finish line like I was at the end of the surgery. I saw myself smiling continuously the closer I got to that date. by all means, it was not an easy journey, but I made the best of it. I prepared it as if it was a pregnancy. I had my suitcase ready with all of the goods needed for surgery. I mentally cleared and freed my head from loss, confusion, anxiety, fear, etc; you name it, I was so ready.

I rolled into surgery in a smile with great confidence, thanks to support from family and close friends. I must say that the support I received on this journey was bigger than me. I will never forget an emotional post shared by a friend on social media about her journey with uterine fibroids. I was in such despair when I read that post. It was a questionable time for me, you know when your mind just starts to shift for no reason, and all you can think of is "Why me?" That was my position when I read that post. It basically entailed of a young lady who could not conceive after a couple of years of marriage, had a doctor's visit, and to her astonishment, it was revealed that she had multiple fibroids. Long story short, her and husband decided that removing the uterine fibroids would be beneficial. About a year later, she finds herself pregnant, now to have two children after an open myomectomy to remove thirty uterine fibroids in her uterus. That postmanaged to have me wipe my tears, and feel that I was not alone. It was such a mixed remarkable feeling, no words can actually explain, but the point is that it gave me hope, courage, and inspiration at that moment, which is exactly what I needed to walk into surgery with my head high. The opportunity to read that post made a major difference in my life. Although, my case was risky, I was confident that my uterus will still be inside of me after I wake up from being under anesthesia.

Sure enough, everything went as planned in God's way. I woke up with a bigger smile than the one I had walking into surgery. Everyone was shocked. I really did not look like I was gone for about two and a half hours. I felt great. My only thought was that " I can't wait to go home to start my new life." I literally found myself counting the days to go home. My release was just after two nights. On that third day, I prepared myself by myself without any staff assistance. I was ready for my new beginning. While I was in recovery, I had many spiritual visitations. I believe and know that God and my ancestors were all present at my surgery assisting and making sure that all goes well. All of the visitations revealed to me that I was not alone. My recovery was challenging, at first, I did not understand it, but one day after deep meditation, I realized the message sent to me. This uterine fibroid journey was not just my journey. I was rather used to go through the ups and down of the journey, lasted long enough through many obstacles to now have a testimony. The testimony is not only for me, it will also for all women struggling with any type of uterine fibroid condition. What a huge responsibility! My first thought was "how is this going to happen?" I was secretive about my condition because that was the way society framed it to be, and I followed the pattern by being silent.

Uterine fibroids was never an acceptable condition. It was not something people talked about. Uterine fibroids were more like a negative stigma put on one's life rather than a blessing. And, I am being challenged to talk about it. The more I suppressed myself, the more pain I experienced. My blood pressure just kept rising. At one point, I thought I was going to have a heart attack. My blood pressure rose to 180/90. I was scared. I ended up in the emergency room for an entire day, just to be told that nothing was wrong. I just need to relax, it is just anxiety, no need for medication. After this episode, I was stern with my communication with God. I was not nice at all. I spoke openly to him like he was my homeboy. "Listen up God, I know very well that you did not bring me this far to get me sick again. Let's just stop all of the nonsense. I am done with having emergency room visits. Enough is enough." I will never forget that amazing loud confident soft voice I heard. The voice said, "Well, ok then, now that you have been delivered, serve my people. That's it!". At that moment, I was in bed, in my room, the television was on at a very low volume, but that voice was loud and clear. I automatically froze. I could not believe the experience I had. It was amazing. This experience brought countless tears, but the importance it that it had me moving in a new direction. As a writer, the best way for me to serve is through my writing. Writing for me is the personal release of emotions. It is a perfect mode of elevation by letting of past fears and obstacles. On that note, I accepted my responsibility to be the chosen one to free God's people with uterine fibroid conditions by sharing my story of hope, courage, and inspiration with a company of women who have suffered, faced and endured all different phases of the condition. That is exactly how *Faces of Uterine Fibroids* was created. Within this anthology, you will find yourself and others in many stories facing many different obstacles, but resulting in the same message of hope, courage, and inspiration. Aside from hope, courage, and inspiration, you will contentment, pride, togetherness, spirituality and women empowerment. This is anthology is about women supporting women. It's a movement.. A movement of enlightenment and encouragement to be a solution for yourself and others. Uterine Fibroids do not always need to be an ugly condition. It does not have to be an issue of abandonment, it can beautiful, just as beautiful as every woman who carries them or not. Uterine fibroids are not lost cases, a miracle comes can happen after surgery. Surgery to remove uterine fibroids or a uterus is not a destitute situation. It is rather a way to a new beginning, a new life with a new ending. The movement with these compilations of stories is to request for more research, more education for a condition which affects everyone, women, men and children. Women are center pillars in all areas of life, if a woman's condition is poor, it becomes a poor reflection on all that she touches. It's a domino effect, so we might as well do our best to obtain in-depth research for the sake of families, workplaces, community organizations, etc. Women are everywhere. We are not going anywhere. Our issues need to address "Awareness of Uterine Fibroids" is a must in schools, especially all girl schools. Why can't this condition be discussed like any other conditions? What is the problem? We all about the vagina, right? So, why can't we talk about an alarmingly concerning condition of the uterus? Well, now the time has come. Hope, courage, and inspiration are here. Women are speaking by stepping out of fear and embarrassment, embracing their God-given condition to heal. In God, with God, there is always a solution. Hope our stories bring great positive transformations to you and your condition.

Martine M. Mayas was born in 1976 in New York to Haitian parents, Jocelyne Mayas and Frantz Mayas. Martine is a Natural Hair Enthusiast and an International Best Selling Author who shares her personal life experiences, style, poise, etiquette, class and sophistication with the world. Contact Martine at email: mindhearthairbodysoul@gmail.com .

We're here for a reason. I believe that reason is to throw little torches out to lead people through the dark.

~Whoopi Goldberg

After your season of suffering, God in all his grace will restore, confirm, strengthen and establish you.

~ 1 Peter 5:10

Pain, Purpose and Promise
Broken to Peace

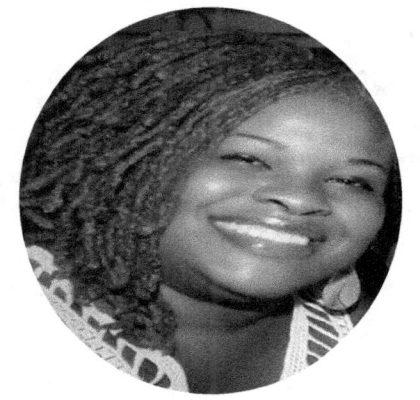

BY: DR. STEPHANIE SHANKLIN

Blessed is she who believed that the Lord would fulfill his promises to her-
~ Luke 1:45

F acing my fibroid reality did not come without a struggle especially when it meant accepting that this journey would lead me down the difficult path to the operating room. There were so many stolen moments from my life as a result of living with fibroids. It robbed me of my freedom of movement, the ability to fully enjoy a holiday or vacation; even simple tasks like driving, walking or being able to take a deep breath became difficult. Living with fibroids also meant breaking promises to my loved ones. My intentions were good

I would make promises when I was feeling good but unfortunately my body would often say no when the time came to keep those promises. I felt broken but through persistence, determination and resilience I realized that I was still in control of my happiness. I relied on my faith and had hope that I would be blessed with peace.

M y fibroid journey started long before the diagnosis or even before I found out what I was experiencing wasn't normal. The pain, pressure, as well as the love hate relationship with my menstrual cycle started almost immediately. I remember the excitement and fear of the first time like it was yesterday but that quickly changed as the symptoms started. My menstrual cycle was always a difficult and painful even as a child; as the years went on and the symptoms worsened I just assumed that this was part of being a woman and that's when suffering in silence became my reality. I accepted that living with the symptoms was real life and a part of me would always be hidden. The heavy periods, cramping, frequent urge to urinate were enough to keep me in the house and in bed for days. My period meant missing school, gym, playing outside, slumber parties and family events but because of the embarrassment hiding the truth also started very early I would lie and say I had a headache or I was on punishment so I could not attend.

As I became older the cost became greater. I would miss important work related meetings and I would have to fight to make the dream of motherhood a reality just to end up missing once in a life time milestones of my children. This life of uncertainty became my normal which I was constantly trying to get used to but I could not accept the toll that this condition was taking on my life as a whole especially on my role as a wife and a mother. The joy of motherhood came with a price because my children had to coexist with my fibroids and after the first two miscarriages I wanted to give up and accept that maybe being a mom would have to be a dream deferred but God would bless me with not one but two beautiful sons. My sons are my greatest blessings & brought so much joy to my life and missing out on life with them just broke my heart. I began praying and impossible became possible. That was the beginning of my foundation of faith. Little did I know that faith would be tested over the years.

This condition impacted every aspect of my life. There was a significant toll emotionally, spiritually, mentally, and on my physical health. I felt lost and alone because in the initial stages of this journey I did not want to talk to anyone or share what I was going through even with my closest family and friends because I felt ashamed and like less of women especially when they my doctors started suggesting a hysterectomy. I wanted to have a normal life free from all the pain and limitations that accompanied my menstrual cycle. I wanted to be able to live without fear of what was to come and I wanted to have an authentic and spontaneous intimate relationship with my husband. I remember crying and when I couldn't cry anymore I started praying and through prayer and spiritual growth I found peace. It wasn't easy I had to face my reality but I also had to believe in God's promise not to leave or forsake me and then and only then did my healing begin. I realized that being a women, wife and mother was about so much more than what was inside of me or whether or not I could have more children. My purpose was rooted deeper than this pain. I had to go through this pain and feeling of brokenness to find my purpose and peace.

Along the way I explored my options watchful waiting, follow-up 1repeat ultrasounds, oral contraceptives, focused ultrasounds, myomectomy, uterine fibroid embolization (UFE), hormone and non-hormonal therapy, as well as a Hysterectomy. The treatment options I tried included watchful waiting and follow-up ultrasounds, and oral contraceptives. In the end after great thought and consideration I choose to have a hysterectomy which would eliminate any possibility of fibroid recurrence but it also meant the loss of reproductive potential and the possibility of early menopause at 30. Early Menopause came with health risks as well. Complications and side effects of a hysterectomy depends on the patient as well as the surgeon and surgical technique used. There a few common complications are infections, bleeding, nerve injury and injury to nearby organs. Additional risks discussed prior to my surgery were: Anesthesia problems, such as breathing or heart problems, Blood clots in the legs or lungs. The consequences of a hysterectomy are real and should be discussed thoroughly before making this life changing decision.

During my recovery, I faced many challenges and side effects which included pain a lot of pain, hot flashes, depression, insomnia, anxiety, irritability, dizziness, nervousness, weight gain, memory lapses, headaches, fatigue, problems with urination, heart palpitations, and heart disease. While this side effects may seem extreme and there were days that I thought maybe I made a mistake but I was confident in my decision to permanently end my fibroid nightmare.

The side effects were difficult to manage and I felt like I was always at the doctor's office. The Physical pain was hard but the emotional pain seemed endless. I had to grieve the loss of my ability to have children which was hard to explain because people thought I should be comforted by the fact that I had two children but healing also meant going through the many stages of grief; I was angry, sad depressed and felt guilty. My family was complete but I didn't feel like a whole woman. But as my life got back to normal and I went back to work the feeling of sadness also began to fade away. Every once and awhile when I would see a baby I would get the tug at my heart but those feelings didn't last long.

Throughout my journey, I discovered many things about myself. I found strength in my faith. I also discovered the importance of hope. During the most difficult times of this journey when it seemed like I couldn't get through this I held on to hope and hope came in many forms. My hope came from just praying or that quiet moment sometimes it came from my sons sharing their day or just a smile from my husband or an encouraging word from a friend. Hope was an important part of my healing because it gave me something to hold on to, look forward to, dream about and work towards. Faith and hope didn't mean everything was great or that life was good but it did give me the courage to look past my pain and see the possibilities in every new day. Hope allowed me to find purpose and peace even during those imperfect moments.

Choosing a hysterectomy was a difficult as it was the most final of the options but I wanted my life back so it was the choice that made the most sense in my life and for my family. I knew that I would have to accept that I would not have any more children but I was blessed with two amazing sons and a loving husband. I was blessed that the experience of a hysterectomy was a unifying experience for my husband and I. We faced it together, talking and listening to one another, discussing our needs, communicating our feelings honestly and with empathy as well as compassion. With the support and love of my family, friend and medical staff I knew I would get through this. I cannot imagine where I would be today if it were not for the handful of friends who have given me a heart full of joy and love throughout this process. They picked me up when I needed it supported me when I thought I couldn't stand and gave me a fresh perspective to face another day. I am blessed that I did not have to go on this journey alone. The surgery was only the beginning, the recovery was hard but I had amazing doctors that prepared me for every step and the most important advise was don't rush it. I took one day at a time and some days I had to take one minute at a time. I listened to my body and was the key to my recovery.

Although my story did not have a fairy tale ending; having a hysterectomy was the best solution for me. God has taken me from broken and in pain to peace and living with purpose which is deeper than my feet could ever wonder. Embracing the hidden, coming out of the dark and realizing that it is important that women have a voice has also allowed me to accept the every aspect of this journey. I found comfort for my heart, spirit and soul within my circle once I shared my pain. My story may have been rooted in pain and with me feeling broken but it is about so much more now; advocating, sharing and sometimes just listening and encouraging other women not to suffer in silence.

Dr. Stephanie Shanklin, Ed.D was raised in Irvington, N.J. She holds a Bachelor's degree in Urban studies and Community Planning from Rutgers University- Camden, a master in Administrative Science from Fairleigh Dickinson University. Stephanie recently earned a Doctorate of Education from Wilmington University. Dr. Shanklin resides in Mt. Royal N.J. where she celebrates each day with her husband, Scott and her sons Ty and Jaylen.

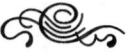

If your actions create a legacy that inspires others to dream more, learn more, do more and become more, then, you are an excellent leader.

~ Dolly Parton

My Journey living with Fibroids
The Courage to Walk in Faith

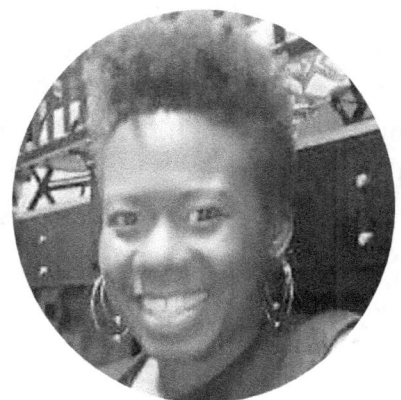

By: Patrice Ross

lthough the first physical indication was a lump I discovered in my pelvic area in November of 2015, as I learned more about fibroid tumors, I am convinced that I had been in the battle far longer than I knew. It wasn't until my annual exam in January 2016 that tumors were confirmed in my uterus via ultrasound. Due to my insurance coverage, it took an additional three month to confirm a benign, fibroid diagnosis. Through the Faces of Uterine Fibroids, I will share with you a synopsis of my journey which will be included in my book coming out in 2017/2018.

L ike most women, single and in my thirties, I was finding myself. I attended church regularly. I was reading self-help books, making vision boards and learning to meditate to get in touch with my inner self so I could navigate being an ambitious single mother. By design, I am a healthy woman. I have an annual medical exam like clockwork each year on or about January 27 th. Never once have I received an abnormal pap smear result. My body, as it should, craves the foods to supplement any deficiencies it experienced. Life was good. If I had to bet money, I believe I can pinpoint the exact time that my true fibroid journey began. I remember scheduling an annual exam and I remember requesting that every possible test be performed. My request should not be considered odd as I had just discovered that most annual exams include very minimal testing though most insurance companies pay for much more as part of their preventative care coverage. I was nervous. My family doctor whom I'd been seeing since I was a teenager had moved out of the city. I was embarrassed because I'd had Bacterial Vaginosis and had never before been to a female OBGYN. My fears were unfounded. She seemed very knowledgeable and has a great bedside manner. It was like having a conversation with one of my best friends. She helped me to feel more aware of my body. I better understood why I battled with Bacterial Vaginosis so often and no longer felt embarrassed. As I awaited my test results, I began to research and change things that affected the ph balance of my vagina. When she called with my results, she had nothing bad to report except for a high level of testosterone. What did that mean? A friend of mine had gotten the same diagnosis and we decided to research it. She also blogged about our discovery at http:www.adornmysmile.com/?=testosterone. It helped me to understand my dominant personality and it also answered my question about why I had the Godforsaken chin hair. With the diagnosis, I was prescribed a birth control pill that would level me out. Sounds easy enough. Unfortunately, that first prescription had me battling nausea. I was given a milder dose that caused sporadic spotting. The final prescription was the last straw as it caused nausea, vomiting and non-stop spotting. I was aggravated with the back and forth doctor's visits and I decided to just stop the treatment altogether. Woe to me, I began to bleed every day. My doctor explained the daily bleeding was caused because of the way I stopped taking the pills and that the bleeding would soon end. The bleeding lasted for about thirty days and my body seemed to go back to what I thought was normal except now my periods because very irregular. Some months were heavy and some light. This was different for me but nothing that I thought was alarming. I was lucky enough not to have too many lifestyle changes during that time of the month. My next exam indicated that while my testosterone levels were back to normal, my iron level was a little low. I was told not to be alarmed because the numbers were not low enough for concern. I appeared to me my normal, energetic, single mother self so I had no complaints.

Later in the year, I had gained the courage to walk away from my job and take a faith walk. My first stop was to return to school. After a few disappointments, I enrolled into a local culinary program. Each day consisted of me standing for at least four hours which could justify my onset of daily exhaustion. Right? After graduating at the top of my class, I began working twelve to fourteen hours at a prestigious country club. That also had to be the explanation of my loss of energy and drive. I had written the vision and made it plain so to give up that easily wasn't in me. I pushed through. When the opportunity permitted I took another leap of faith and went into business for myself as a Personal Chef. The hours on my feet during each event would clock well over fourteen hours. The only difference was the frequency of events was weekly compared to daily. At the time of my next annual exam, my insurance had changed and I was now being seen by a primary care physician. My iron levels were lower than before and was diagnosed with anemia. Knowing what I now know about eating healthy I requested to be allowed a natural approach to treatment. She agreed to give me a month to take a natural approach before she would impose any medical treatment. Through research and experimentation, I increased my natural iron intake. My energy appeared to be somewhat restored but I was not back to normal. When I returned for my follow-up there was no significant change. I was prescribed to an iron supplement. I was stubborn. I chose healthy eating and would show her by my next annual exam that natural, healthy eating was better than drugs.

Laying in bed one day, I noticed a golf ball sized lump on my right pelvis. It moved and was tender to the touch. I scheduled an appointment immediately. I was reprimanded about not taking my iron prescription and sent off for an ultrasound. The ultrasound revealed four masses in my uterus. My primary care physician would have refer me to an OBGYN for further test and a proper diagnosis. Though she was convinced it was fibroid tumors, which was causing the iron deficiency. Now it was imperative that I took my prescribed iron supplement, no excuses. I then had to wait for three months before a doctor who would take my insurance had a an available appointment. Other than the anemia I didn't have any other symptoms. Tired or not, I always pushed forward, but I will admit some days were unbearable. I was afraid that due to some personal issues in my life my depression had set in. I was mentally tired; Tired of being a single mother and tired of having to be so strong. I felt like my testimony of faith was slowly fading. I began to question every decision I had made to walk in faith and pursue my dreams. Business as a Personal Chef had slowed down but so had my motivation to even market or promote my business. My menstrual cycles began to be heavy and longer. Being unsure of my true diagnosis was adding to the stress which in turn was adding to the onset of symptoms. My life was changing rapidly. I was turning forty in May. I had planned my 2016 to be a year of celebration and testimony. Instead, I lost a relationship and a few friends, plus lack of business begin to threaten eviction and repossession. At what I would consider a very low point in my life I had to suck it all up and get a job. Aside from an issue of pride, working came easy to me. I often excelled in most tasks I took on. I signed on at a temporary staffing agency as a Line Cook. My second assignment became steady. I was a Floating Line Cook. I would train on every station of the cafeteria at a local business park, act as the fill-in for the permanent staff going on vacation or sick leave. I absolutely hated this job. Never in my life had I worked a job with staff who bullied the management and clients who treated staff as servants. I showed up every day though. I had to pray before I walked in each day. My symptoms began to increase. My appointment was coming up but not soon enough. Soon my monthly menstrual cycle turned into a daily routine. It wouldn't go away. I attributed it to the tumors and standing on my feet for eight to ten hours per day. Once I finally made it to my doctor's visit, I was changing my pad every hour. I was messing up my clothes at work almost weekly. The pressure of the staff and clients wasn't helping, so I QUIT! Not like I had never quit a job before, but not like this. I always did it the right way. Gave my proper two-week notice and had another job in place. Not this time, I no called no showed and called the staffing agency by the end of the day and told them I wasn't going back. I even refused reassignment.

All the while I thought it to be depression not knowing the tumors were taking control of my life. Aside from not being able to work, I also couldn't maintain a social life due to fear of having an accident in public. Any chance of a sexual relationship was absolutely out of the question. Thankfully, I walked into the office of a OBGYN who was very confident and familiar with fibroid tumors. His first order of business was to stop the bleeding. Two weeks later I would need to return for a biopsy and go over options. I, on the other hand, I felt so empowered with an actual diagnosis. Now I could google and establish my own healing process. I filled the prescription and it stopped the bleeding overnight. That coupled with the iron supplement I was feeling much better. Euphoria. The following week I signed on with another staffing agency for a position as an administrative assistant. I was back working within a week. My moods were better. I had two additional doctor appointments before we would discuss options and excruciating biopsy and an additional ultrasound. All seemed well in the world until I began to have an allergic reaction to the hormone pill prescribed. I stopped immediately but didn't get a new prescription for about two weeks. This, of course, meant two weeks of heavy bleeding, that actually turned into continued bleeding right up until the date of my surgery. The new prescription was a lower dosage of a hormone to help stop the bleeding. Unfortunately, it only lightened the flow.

On decision day, my doctor, wanted my answer to his golden question, "Do you want any more children?" Well, my logic is that although I am forty and have a 15-year old son, I've never been married. Therefore, if my knight in shining armor comes through and whisks me away, I can still give him an heir to the throne. Not to mention, I enjoy having all my body parts. He explained to me how the myomectomy procedure would work and sent me to scheduling. Yes, I know, Not many options. At the same time, I was only interested in any option that would make the bleeding stop. It wouldn't be for three more months before I would even be scheduled to have the procedure completed.

Be it the stigma or reputation of fibroid tumors among my family and friends, I was either told to leave them alone or get a full hysterectomy. No one seemed to understand the angst I felt. The constant mood swings, bleeding and tiredness was really controlling my life. Even now I feel like my face aged a lot throughout this past year. Everyone felt I should just be sure to keep pads at my disposal when I have time get some rest and swelled bellies came with age. I researched all I could to avoid the surgery. Most natural remedies and solutions called for eight to nine months to see good results. I could not fathom bleeding for another year. I stumbled upon a support group on Facebook that really helped me to better understand what I was dealing with. It was refreshing to find so many women who could relate to my symptoms. Not to mention the multiple options I truly had. Coupled with prayer, I was ready to do whatever I needed to do to live better. Instead of dreading an upcoming surgery, I began to look at it as rebirth and restoration. I saw God cleaning my womb and preparing me for my knight in shining armor. I was being made whole. I remember reading somewhere that each tumor was a possible representation of stress you were experiencing in life. As I admitted earlier 2016 was rather stressful. During my ultrasounds, it was reported that 4 fibroid tumors filled my uterus. One which was rapidly growing and causing me the bulk of my symptoms. My stomach was the size of that of a woman who was four months pregnant. I became less active not only due to lack of energy but due to my self-esteem diminishing. Having culinary knowledge I began to research foods to eliminate and add to my diet to help me with my diagnosis. I also leaned on the knowledge of my natural guru and herbalist Stacey Smithe of Sweet Naturals, LLC. She initially gave me a regimen to help shrink the fibroid tumors over a course of six to eight months. With the increase of symptoms, she encouraged me to move forward with my myomectomy with plans to utilize the regimen afterward to help maintain a healthy uterus. I have since had my myomectomy. Instead of four fibroid tumors, my doctor retrieved nine fibroid tumors. Instead of three to four weeks of out of work, I was out of work for six weeks and am still somewhat recovering. My number one priority is eliminating all stress. Secondly, I am trying to streamline my diet. I am making great strides. I have eliminated soda. I am minimizing sugar and starch while increasing my fruits and vegetables. I juice a combination of fruits and vegetables at least three days per week to avoid the return of fibroid tumors. I am encouraging women I know personally to monitor and maintain a healthy body, especially their uterus. As mentioned earlier, I will release a novel/cookbook combination 'Issue of Blood' which will inspire healthy eating on a fibroid journey. I am more empowered than I have ever felt in any other life event. I hope that as you read you to feel empowered to overcome our journey.

Patrice Ross, Mother, Entrepreneur, Author, Chief, CEO and Chief Executive Officer at Sincerely Patrice, Studied Culinary Arts at Virginia College in Jacksonville Lives in Jacksonville, Florida, Fibroids warrior

Sometimes it's the smallest decisions that can change your life forever

~ Keri Russell

What You Don't Know Can Hurt You

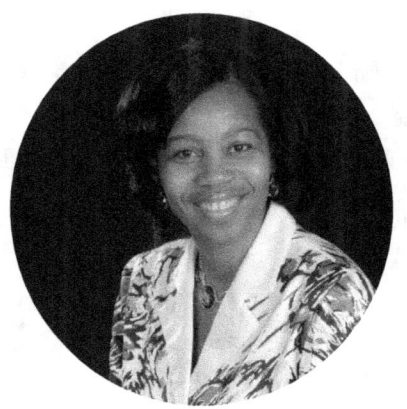

BY: ANDREA E. MONROE

My involvement in the book that you now hold in your hands came from a one-one-one conversation I had with Martine Mayas. She is the Powerful and Passionate Fibroid Warrior that God used to undertake this much-needed topic and project.

So, I would be the one who had two fibroid surgeries and never questioned how this could happen to me or why this happened to me. I was told I had them and they needed to come out if I wanted to be able to conceive a child. They were not a hindrance to me or so I thought. My chapter is dedicated to the women and young ladies who may or may not know that you have fibroids.

If you know you have them…ask questions. If you do not know or you are unsure, please ask questions. Especially, if you have heavy and painful menses along with anemia.

Now my Fibroid Warrior story:

As a teenager, when my menses started it was VERY heavy and painful. My mother could not believe how heavy it was. I started off with Tampax tampons. The pain that I would experience was horrible. I thought as I got older it would get better but it did not. It became worse but it never got better prior to my first surgery. Motrin 800mg and my heating pad became my best friends. I would take two pills every four hours and they would not take the pain away. However, they would take the edge off for me to be able to bear it.

I remember being in high school and bleeding through my clothes. Can you say embarrassed? I was the last one to leave the class. I had a jacket that I wrapped around my waist to conceal the blood. I also remember the blood spot on my desk seat. Which I tried to wipe up. We had the wooden desks during that timeframe. I went to the bathroom and tried to clean myself up but the more I tried the more I bled. I finally went to the office to have them call my mother. She was a God send to me.

That day, I was taught 2 valuable lessons. First, I needed to have ample supply of tampons and pads with me ALL the time. Second, my cycle was not regimented to the normal 21 – 28 day cycle menses. My menses had a mind and cycle all its own.

At the age of 18, I joined the military. I was introduced to a world of many different kinds of people. They were like me and not like me at the same time. Different backgrounds, skin tones, dialects, and cultures. At the beginning of my new journey, I was dealing with something that was unique to JUST ME. We are talking late 80's and early 90's. I was the only one like me. So, I learned to live a VERY lonely and painful existence. I felt alone, lonely, unloved and unlovable.

I remember having to leave work because my pain was so bad. They sent me to Sick Call which was the equivalent of primary care. The doctor talked to me and I told her I had heavy menses with pain associated with it every month. I was given Birth Control pills and was told they would help with the heavy bleeding. During this appointment, I was also told I was severely anemic. I was also given pain meds and iron pills.

A memory came back to me as I am writing my chapter. I saw myself in the fetal position on my bed in excruciating pain. I was holding my stomach and praying for God to help me. This was NOT abnormal for me. This was a normal part of my menstrual cycles. I had gotten used to the pain and I was "the only one" going through this. My mother never dealt with this sort of pain or heavy bleeding during her menses. My friends were not dealing with this. So, I had no one to turn to. Therefore, I learned early on that I was supposed to just deal with this pain and keep it moving. This was just the way I was designed. I was one who suffered in silence. You may be dealing with and thinking the same thing but there is hope and you are holding it in your hands.

As I am writing, the thought just hit me that we as women can get used to this and we think it is just the way we are or it is the way we were designed. We can blame ourselves or God. But the thing we can do immediately is make an appointment with our GYN to ask questions and get some answers. While you wait for your appointment do something else for you. Do an internet search for uterine fibroids. There is a wealth of information out there if you will look. There are more women just like you than you realize. This book you hold in your hands is just a handful of us. **If you are not dealing with it but know a woman who is bless her with this book.**

I had experienced almost ALL of the symptoms for uterine fibroids but did not know it. These are the symptoms I experienced:

Heavy menses – going through almost two boxes of tampons and pads each month. If I had the foresight to invested in Playtex tampons I would be a rich girl. It would be a money back program. When I spent money, I would receive a dividend.

Severe pain – pain that would shut me down for days at a time. This pain would have me in the fetal position more times than I could count.

Bloating – feelings of being fat all the time when I weighed between 110 and 130

Painful sexual intercourse – sex was always a chore because it was painful for me

Difficulty getting pregnant – I wanted children but did not know the fibroids were blocking that from happening

Anemia – extreme blood loss due to my menses hurt me. I was weak and cold all the time.

Social Barriers -Can't talk about it because no one was going through what I was going through. Therefore, they would not understand.

Depression – I was depressed and did not even know it until I came out of it and began to look back over my life.

Mood Swings – I would be up one minute, tears the next, and down the next. I was on a continuous roller coaster of emotions. I would just have outburst for no apparent reason.

• **Side Note:** As I look back over my Fibroid journey that I did not even know I was on. The first doctor to point out or even use the term fibroids was an African American female. Prior to that every doctor had been Caucasian both male and female. Don't settle for one opinion get another. Remember, you have to take care of you. You are your own best advocate.

As my title states, what you don't know can hurt you. I separated from the military after 15 years and still had the painful cycles and heavy menses. In 2009, I went to see a new doctor and during our initial consultation she asked me had I ever been diagnosed with fibroids. I responded no. What is that? She continued to explain that they were tumors in the uterus and usually benign. They can cause heavy bleeding during menses, severe pain, and anemia. All of these I was experiencing. So, she sent me for blood tests and a pelvis MRI. The blood test showed I was anemic and the MRI showed I did have uterine fibroids. I had multiple ones. My uterus measured 13 x 10 x 10 cm. The dominant one measured 7.3 x 6.0 x 7.4. It took up over half of my uterus by itself. There were others that were 2 cm and smaller in size. I was shocked as she told me.

We discussed next steps which were surgery options. She asked if I wanted children. I responded yes. She said you will want to choose the laparoscopic myomectomy because it will leave your female reproductive system in place. This was scary for me because I had never had any type of surgery before. She said it would be outpatient surgery. This means I was admitted to the hospital and had surgery. Once I was able to tolerate the pain and urinate then I was released. I left the same day.

My first ever surgery:

2010 - Laparoscopic Myomectomy

- Left my female organs intact
- 3 bikini cut incisions
- 4 weeks to recover for me. (norm then 4 - 6 weeks; now 2 weeks)
- outpatient surgery.

After my surgery, my cycle decreased to 3 – 5 days and there was little to no pain during my menses. My menses was not heavy at all. I also gained a regulated menses which I had never experienced before. I had entered a new world and was overjoyed to be a part of it. I had no idea women could actually live like this. My attitude changed and I did not even realize it. My focus became more clear. I saw myself from a different perspective. I saw me with new eyes. I went on a shopping spree with just me. I picked out colors: pink, yellow, vibrant blues, red, orange, etc. My previous wardrobe consisted of black, browns, and navy blues. I had a new lease on life. I knew that I wanted more out of life than I currently had. I had taken off my mask.

I just thought about my wardrobe and how it reflected how I was feeling or who I had become. The navy blues, browns, and blacks could conceal the blood if I had an "accident". The embarrassment from high school had followed me into adulthood. I never realized that until just now. How are you feeling and who have you become in your fibroid battle? Is it the person you desire to be?

The surgery and recovery time caused me to own up to my truths. Did I want to continue to play the victim in my own life? Did I want to continue to be in a loveless marriage? I owned up to two major mistakes I had made. First, I was broken and needed to be married to fix me. Second, I married the wrong person. I was gaining clarity as I walked through the process of recovery. I prayed about the surgery and I only asked God to let me wake up after the surgery. HE did that gave me soooooooooo much more.

As you hold this book in your hands maybe you are dealing with life from a victim mentality instead of a victor mentality. You are going through the motions of existing but you are not living your life. God made you wonderfully complex (Psalm 139:14). You are unique, beautiful, amazing, and lovely in your own right. You are the daughter of the King of Kings and Lord of Lords. You are more than you have become.

I had to be taught how to look at and love me just the way I was. For me, I needed hope and my hope was found in Jesus Christ. Prior to I was just a shell of who I was actually created by God to be.

B eing happily remarried, I wanted children. So, we sought help. I was referred to a Reproductive Endocrinologist for testing and was sent for another MRI. I was told the fibroids had come back. I thought, I was fine because they had been previously removed. But they were back. I had noticed a heavier than usual menses and more cramping but because it was not at the level it was before I disregarded the same symptoms. I was told if we wanted children I would have to have another surgery. My husband and I discussed it. He said it was ultimately my decision since it was my body. So, I decided to go through with the surgery. This time it was a robotic assisted surgery.

Second Surgery:
2015 – Robotic Assisted Myomectomy surgery
- left my female organs intact
- done specifically to remove fibroids so I could have children
- more involved due to a hematoma in my side developed during surgery

After the second surgery, I woke up in a hospital room and was told I would be staying for a couple days. The couple turned into 4 days. They could not get my blood pressure to rise. This meant every time I tried to stand I would pass out. They said I did not lose a lot of blood during surgery so the doctors were confused as to why my blood pressure was so low.

After many tests and blood transfusions I was allowed to leave the hospital with my wonderful husband and mother-in-love. She was a God send. After the second surgery, I was told that my diet has a lot to do with the growth of fibroids. I don't remember this talk after my first surgery but I took note and asked the questions after the second surgery.

I was told caffeine is a big advocate for fibroids. I loved chocolate especially Hot chocolate and Oreo cookie ice cream. But I had to either give it up or face the alternative for me. It was a no-brainer. I love tea but I only drink decaffeinated teas now. (You can Google "foods to avoid with fibroids".) Since signing on to this project I have learned through speaking with Martine and belonging to our closed Facebook group that there are many other options than just surgery. This was my path but it does not have to be yours unless absolutely necessary. There are herbal ways to shrink and get rid of fibroids so you can have a more normal life.

Please hear me **there are other options than just surgery**. The other options like nutrition and herbs were NOT presented to me. I do not blame my doctors. I don't even blame myself. But as the old saying goes: "when you know better, you do better." You cannot stay stuck in the world of what ifs or would have, could have, should have been. Choose to move on into what you know right now as a result of the new information you now hold in your hands.

You can look at it as new or confirmation of something that has been spoken to or tugging at you. Now that you have been armed with the information:

Will you choose to take off the mask and get help?

You can choose to continue in your current path. Or you can choose to be your own best advocate when it comes to helping you turn your fibroid walk into a fibroid warrior stance.

Andrea E. Monroe, a writer, blogger, an encourager, and speaker who focuses on setting the captives free in others. She is the Founder and President of Women of Valour: Releasing the Spirit Within and Warriors for Christ Ministries. She has a Master's degree in the darkness that keeps women bound to their past and even their present. Her platform is No More Masks. She desires to help women remove their masks and see themselves for who they were actually created to be. She accomplishes this by being transparent and revealing her own masks. She is also a loving wife who is married to Carlton L. Monroe.

UTERINE FIBROID REGROWTH PREVENTION

CHERISH™

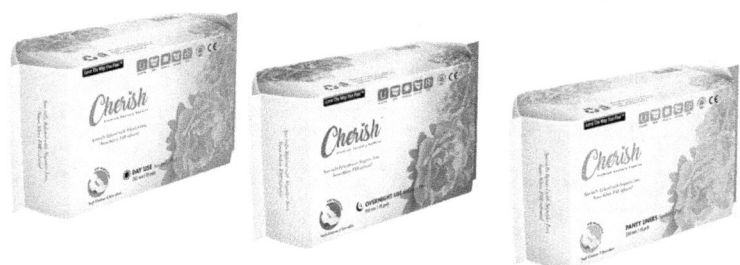

CHERISH™ DAY USE PREMIUM SANITARY NAPKINS

Ladies, this is what you have been waiting for! Cherish Premium Daily Use Pads are designed with 8 layers to keep you feeling fresh, dry and protect you for hours on your busiest days. Cherish Premium Day Pads, while ultra-thin, include a super-absorbent and safe polymer that is up to 10 timeAs more absorbent than conventional pads and holds more than 300 times its own weight in liquid!

The unique negative ion strip has many proven health benefits including possibly reducing pain and inflammation and may help to neutralize unwanted odors. Now you can maintain an active, carefree lifestyle during that most sensitive time of the month. With Cherish premium pads, you're going to Love the Way You Feel™.

HTTP://WWW.NSPIRENETWORK.COM/MARTINE

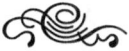

Thank you for Reading!

*Please add a short review on Amazon
and let me know what you thought!*

#1 Author Martine M. Mayas

www.amazon.com/author/martinemayas

Mayas & Company, LLC
Visionary & Creative Consultant

#1 International Best Selling Author

email: mindhearthairbodysoul@gmail.com

www.amazon.com/author/martinemayas

Faces of Uterine Fibroids Fashion Corner

www.cafepress.com/fouf

Faces of Uterine Fibroids invites every reader and supporter to join their group at:

www.facebook.com/groups/facesofuterinefibroids

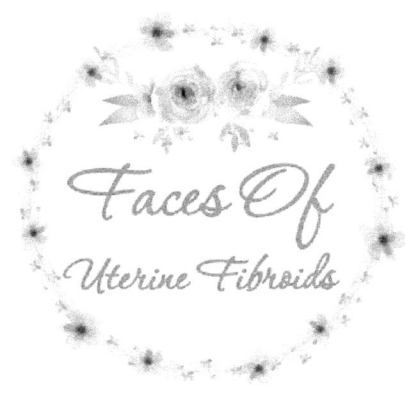

FACES OF UTERINE FIBROIDS

FASHION CORNER

Please visit my online shop!

Great gifts for yourself and friends. You'll find unique merchandise with my art on t-shirts, sweatshirts, mugs, stickers, and more.

WWW.CAFEPRESS.COM/FOUF

www.ingramcontent.com/pod-product-compliance
Lightning Source LLC
Chambersburg PA
CBHW071235280526
45787CB00002B/938